How to fight cardiovascular disease naturally

By

Joseph Moshood

Gladstar gifted and talented educational centre. A

registered member of Nigeria Network of Non-Government

Organizations

Follow us or our Executive Director at www.facebook.com/moshood.joseph, www.facebook.com/gladstargiftedandtalentededucationalcentre,http://ng.linkein.com/pub/joseph-moshood/19/a91/484, www.twitter.com/jmgladstar, www.twitter.com/GGiftedEducate, www.slideshare.net/jmgladstar

Gladstar gifted and talented educational centre- committed to education for sustainable development. For any enquiry or sponsorship, call +2348059879785 or email jmgladstar@gmail.com

Table of content

Follow us or our Executive Director at
www.facebook.com/moshood.joseph,
www.facebook.com/gladstargiftedandtalentededucationalce ntre,http://ng.linkein.com/pub/joseph-moshood/19/a91/484,
www.twitter.com/jmgladstar,
www.twitter.com/GGiftedEducate,
www.slideshare.net/jmgladstar

INTRODUCTION

In the past, we felt that we have low incidence of heart disease. This perception of low incidence is was mainly because it was under-diagnosed especially in developing countries. Some people inform you of a neighbor or relative who suddenly slump and die while walking by the road, watching a football match or climbing staircase; such a person die of heart failure in most case but there

was no proof to substantiate it then. Angiograms

are now revealing that there are more people

suffering from coronary heart disease.

 The pattern of heart disease in Nigeria and other

developing countries is changing due to our

adoption of western type of food and lifestyle.

There is a lot of stress due to the economic

pressure in most of our cities which tend to

increase the work-hour and reduce leisure and rest.

All these are some of the risk factors for heart

disease. Heart disease is on the increase in our

cities and we need to fight it so that we can live

longer.

 The cost and emotional implication of heart

disease on the patients is worth a fortune. In

Ghana, the cost of a heart valve operation for a

Ghanaian is $5000 and $10000 for foreigners. In

Nigeria, a heart valve operation will cost about 1.5

million naira. Even if the money is available, the

emotional agonies that the patients will be passing

through are more dreadful than death.

Gladstar gifted and talented educational centre- committed to education for sustainable development. For any enquiry or sponsorship, call +2348059879785 or email jmgladstar@gmail.com

With all these in view, you need to do all that you can to fight heart disease and save yourself from many troubles. The Lord declared that my people perish because they lack knowledge. This is a mighty weapon that we want to put in your hand and you must use to save yourself from the evil around. Cardiac attack, blockage and failure are heart diseases that you must nip in the buck to avoid the calamities imbedded in them.

STRESS AND CARDIOVASCULAR DISEASE

Stress is any strain or interference that disturbs the functioning of a person. Whenever you are troubled by the situation around you and you feel helpless about it, then you are stressed out. Human beings tend to respond to physical and psychological stress with a combination of psychic and physiological defenses. For every action, there is equal and opposite reaction. You are bound to

act irrationally when you feel stressed and you

could put up enough defenses in term of a smile,

egocentric display or diversion techniques.

  Stress is an unavoidable effect of living and is an

especially complex concept in modern

technological society. The demand of our day-to-

day job deals with deadlines to meet, a bus to

board, and a delay task to accomplish and so on.

There is little or no doubt that a person's success

or failure in controlling potentially stressful

situations can have profound effect on his ability to

function. You must see yourself as the person in

control before you can achieve your desired

success and suppress the stressful situations around

you.

The ability to cope with stress has been

emphasized in psychosomatic research.

Researchers have reported a statistical link

between coronary heart disease and individuals

exhibiting stressful behavioral patterns like

impatience, sense of time urgency, hard driving

Gladstar gifted and talented educational centre- committed to education for sustainable development. For any enquiry or sponsorship, call +2348059879785 or email jmgladstar@gmail.com

competitiveness and pre-occupation with

vocational and related deadlines.

Various strategies have been successful in

treating psychological and physiological stress.

Moderate stress may be relieved by

1. Exercise and any type of meditation.

2. Try to think outside the box.

3. Take a scriptural verse related to that

   problem, read it out to you and think of how

   to use it in view of the situation around.

Severe stress may require psychotherapy to

uncover and work through the underlying

causes. A form of behavior therapy known as

biofeedback can be used to assist a person.

Biofeedback is information supplied

instantaneously about an individual's

psychological process. Data such as

cardiovascular activity (blood pressure and

heart rate), temperate, brain waves or muscle

tension is monitored electronically and returned

or 'fed back' to that person through a gauge on a meter, a light or sound. With these, an individual learns to control his body reaction to stress.

Sometimes a change of environment or living situation may produce therapeutic result. Personally, I found out that music therapy is also effective or all type of stress. After a busy day's work, listening to a solemn music can drain out all stress in you.

Hypertension and Cardiovascular disease

Hypertension, also called High blood pressure is becoming the feature of at least ten percent o our working population. No man can boast of being immunized from this condition because it is promoted by situations around you which lack control over as well as those that you can control. High blood pressure is a condition in which the blood pressure is abnormally high in the arteries or veins. Most physicians consider the blood pressure of healthy adult to be around 120/80.

When the blood vessels lose their flexibility, or the muscle surrounding them force their contraction whereby the heart may pump more forcefully to move the same amount of blood through the narrowed vessels into the capillaries and thereby increasing the blood pressure. If this continues over time, this high blood pressure or hypertension can damage the arterioles (the small terminal of an artery that ends in the capillaries) in such organs as the liver, kidney or brain and can

weaken the overworked heart.

 High blood pressure is known as silent killer

because it can be present or years without

perceptible system. It is usually detected by a

routine blood pressure test and in view of that, it is

advisable to regularly go for routine blood pressure

test. The earlier you discovered it and start

managing it effectively, the longer you will live.

 You need to identify the causes and endeavor to

minimize or eradicate those ones that you can. It

Gladstar gifted and talented educational centre- committed to education for sustainable development. For any enquiry or sponsorship, call +2348059879785 or email jmgladstar@gmail.com

was discovered that stressful situations that deals with deadlines and impatience can lead to hypertension. This is because the urge to achieve a goal at all cost will make the demand of blood inflow by the brain higher and thereby the heart will be pressurized to release it faster. If you are working under such condition daily and for longer, you need to change your career, work post or even your employment status so that you can manage this condition that had been inflicted upon you.

Pregnancy and use of oral contraceptives can also lead to high blood pressure. If you don't space your children for at least two years, it may lead to hypertension. This is in view of the pressure on the heart is higher when pregnant and this may not lead to high blood pressure in most cases but sometime does. Use of oral contraceptives especially by overweight ladies can lead to high blood pressure. It is therefore suggested that such women should use other method of family planning.

You are likely to have hypertension, if there is a trait of hypertension in your lineage. Apart from this, there are some unknown origins of hypertension. The narrowing of the aorta of the heart by fat/cholesterol deposit can also lead to hypertension. This is common among those that are overweight.

Despite the fatal consequences of high blood pressure, like congestive heart failure, kidney failure or stroke, if untreated; the condition responds well to medicine and other therapeutic measures. In its milder forms, hypertension is

usually treated with a self-help regimen that

include a no-salt diet, a weight reducing diet, a

decrease in or cessation of smoking, mild exercise

and the avoidance of or more successful coping

with stressful situations.

If a self-help program does not help lower your

blood pressure, the physician will usually prescribe

diuretics or sympathetic nerve blockers and use of

drugs for severe hypertension.

Smoking and heart disease

Smoking is the inhaling and exhaling o the fumes of burning plant materials especially tobacco, from a cigarette, cigar or pipe. The American Indians used tobacco in ceremonials (e.g. the smoking of the pipe of peace) and believed it possessed medical properties.

Despite social, religious and current medical arguments against the use of tobacco, the habit has become worldwide. Nicotine and related

alkaloids furnish the narcotic effects of the

substance. Nicotine, the brain poison found in

tobacco, is one of the most deadly poisons

known to man. The first use of tobacco brings

on the symptoms of poisoning like nausea,

dizziness and vomiting. As the body becomes

accustomed to it, these symptoms disappear,

but the poisoning of the body continues.

Smoking is also a prime risk factor in

cardiovascular diseases. Nicotine contracts the

blood vessels and do release hormones that

raise the blood pressure. Both effects could

have an adverse effect on the heart. Smokers

have distinctly higher levels of carbon (11)

oxide in their blood than non-smokers. Carbon

(11) oxide readily combines with hemoglobin,

causing many physiological effects. One of

these physiological effects is a decrease in the

amount of hemoglobin available to carry

oxygen and a resulting increase in the affinity

for oxygen that is available. It has been

revealed that even small amount of carbon (11)

oxide decrease the exercise ability of

individuals with known coronary artery disease.

It is not an easy task to break away from

tobacco smoking but it is quite possible. The

following steps will help you to stay away from

smoking habit and live longer:

1. You must make a firm

decision to stop smoking.

2. You must disassociate with

tobacco users immediately.

3. You must use water and unfermented juices regularly. These who have broken the habit reported that they drink 8-10 glasses of water a day.

4. You must take diet made of mainly fruits and protein from legumes and wheat. Don't take fried and greasy food.

5. You must avoid meat, tea, spicy foods and coffee because they

Gladstar gifted and talented educational centre- committed to education for sustainable development. For any enquiry or sponsorship, call +2348059879785 or email jmgladstar@gmail.com

are irritants that will excite the

nervous system and cause it to

cry out for nicotine again.

6. Engage in physical exercise

along with deep breathing

exercise during waking hours to

enhance blood flow.

7. Never yield to any temptation to

try smoking again.

8. Remember that smoking

darkens the lungs and heart

Gladstar gifted and talented educational centre- committed to education for sustainable development. For any enquiry or sponsorship, call +2348059879785 or email jmgladstar@gmail.com

making it to overwork. When you smoke, your heart has to work harder to pump blood through your blood vessels which had become smaller. Live and enjoy the fruit of your labour by saying NO to smoking.

Gladstar gifted and talented educational centre- committed to education for sustainable development. For any enquiry or sponsorship, call +2348059879785 or email jmgladstar@gmail.com

Infections and cardiovascular disease

The most common infection that can lead to heart disease is rheumatic fever. It is like malaria but not the same as malaria. It symptoms like sore throat, joint pains, running nose, cold and cough. Rheumatic fever is common in children and adolescents. Its cause is uncertain, but it has been found that the condition develops after infection by certain streptococcus bacteria, particularly after

Follow us or our Executive Director at www.facebook.com/moshood.joseph, www.facebook.com/gladstargiftedandtalentededucationalce ntre,http://ng.linkein.com/pub/joseph-moshood/19/a91/484, www.twitter.com/jmgladstar, www.twitter.com/GGiftedEducate, www.slideshare.net/jmgladstar

throat infection. It is believed that rheumatic fever

is an allergic reaction to streptococcus bacteria.

The most serious aspect of rheumatic fever is its

possible effect on the heart. In some cases the heart

becomes inflamed. This makes the heart valves not

to unction properly and can only be corrected

through surgery.

Rest is of primary importance in the treatment o

rheumatic fever. You should promptly treat any

throat sore that you experience with antibiotics

Gladstar gifted and talented educational centre- committed to education for sustainable development. For any enquiry or sponsorship, call +2348059879785 or email jmgladstar@gmail.com

prescribed by medical personnel so that it may not

degenerate to heart disease.

Follow us or our Executive Director at
www.facebook.com/moshood.joseph,
www.facebook.com/gladstargiftedandtalentededucationalce
ntre,http://ng.linkein.com/pub/joseph-moshood/19/a91/484,
www.twitter.com/jmgladstar,
www.twitter.com/GGiftedEducate,
www.slideshare.net/jmgladstar

Natural foods and cardiovascular disease

Throughout the last decade, there had been much inquiry into the subject of fats in the diet. It has been determined that the blood cholesterol level rises when the intake of saturated fats is greater than that of unsaturated fats. You can reduce the cholesterol level in your blood and retard the growth of arteriosclerosis by including largely unsaturated fats in your diet. Saturated fats are from animal sources(like meat, milk, eggs and cream) while unsaturated fats are coconut oil, vegetable oil, corn oil, fish oil and safflower oil.

It has been discovered that a vegetarian's diet is best for promoting long life. A research finding revealed that deaths by heart attack or stroke among vegetarians occurred fifteen years later than such death among the general population. To live longer, make food rich in unsaturated fats instead of saturated fats your choice and consider the following natural foods that will strengthen your

heart as part of your meal daily:

1. Onion: A good blood medicine; lowers

   blood cholesterol; thin blood; retards

   clotting in the heart; regulates blood

   sugar and relieves bronchial congestion.

2. Melon: lowers the rate of lung cancer;

   rich in beta-carotene; also an effective

   blood thinner.

Gladstar gifted and talented educational centre- committed
to education for sustainable development. For any enquiry
or sponsorship, call +2348059879785 or email
jmgladstar@gmail.com

3. Mushroom: lowers blood cholesterol;

    thins blood and stimulates the immune

    system.

4. Lemon/lime: helps lowers blood

    cholesterol.

5. Cherry: an excellent blood builder.

6. Carrots: lowers blood cholesterol,

    prevents constipation, cut down chances

    of contacting cancer of the pancreas.

7. Garlic: It is used to emulsify cholesterol

    and loosen it from the arterial walls. It

Follow us or our Executive Director at
www.facebook.com/moshood.joseph,
www.facebook.com/gladstargiftedandtalentededucationalce
ntre,http://ng.linkein.com/pub/joseph-moshood/19/a91/484,
www.twitter.com/jmgladstar,
www.twitter.com/GGiftedEducate,
www.slideshare.net/jmgladstar

also stimulates activity of the digestive organs.

8. Egg plants/Garden eggs: helps protect the arteries from cholesterol damage; for balancing diets; blocks certain viruses and cause causing agents.

9. Walnut: Rich in fibre and vitamins; lowers blood cholesterol and regulates blood sugar.

10. Soya bean: used to reduce blood cholesterol; regulates blood sugar, the

functions of the colon and prevent bowel problems.

11. Orange: protects the arteries from diseases, fights arterial plague and lower blood cholesterol.

12. Olive: good for heart diseases; thin blood, lowers blood pressure and reduce cholesterol.

13. Honey: has some disinfectant properties or wound and sores; recommended for

throat sores, calm nerves, relief of

asthma and induces sleep.

14. Grapes: A good blood purifier and also

good for catarrh conditions.

15. Apple: keeps the cardiovascular system

healthy by stabilizing blood sugar and

lowering blood cholesterol.